Child Survival Profile: Cambodia

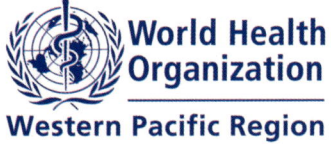

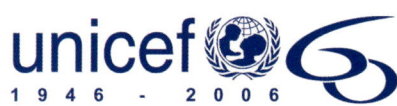

WHO Library Cataloguing in Publication Data
Child Survival Profile: Cambodia.

1. Child survival. 2. Child mortality. 3. Child welfare. 4. Cambodia

ISBN 978 92 9061 224 7   (NLM Classification: **WA 320**)

© World Health Organization 2007
All rights reserved.

The designations employed and the presentation of the material in this publication do not imply the expression of any opinion whatsoever on the part of the World Health Organization concerning the legal status of any country, territory, city or area or of its authorities, or concerning the delimitation of its frontiers or boundaries. Dotted lines on maps represent approximate border lines for which there may not yet be full agreement.

The mention of specific companies or of certain manufacturers' products does not imply that they are endorsed or recommended by the World Health Organization in preference to others of a similar nature that are not mentioned. Errors and omissions excepted, the names of proprietary products are distinguished by initial capital letters.

The World Health Organization does not warrant that the information contained in this publication is complete and correct and shall not be liable for any damages incurred as a result of its use.

Publications of the World Health Organization can be obtained from Marketing and Dissemination, World Health Organization, 20 Avenue Appia, 1211 Geneva 27, Switzerland (tel: +41 22 791 2476; fax: +41 22 791 4857; email: bookorders@who.int). Requests for permission to reproduce WHO publications, in part or in whole, or to translate them – whether for sale or for noncommercial distribution – should be addressed to Publications, at the above address (fax: +41 22 791 4806; email: permissions@who.int). For WHO Western Pacific Regional Publications, request for permission to reproduce should be addressed to Publications Office, World Health Organization, Regional Office for the Western Pacific, P.O. Box 2932, 1000, Manila, Philippines, Fax. No. (632) 521-1036, email: publications@wpro.who.int

Table of Contents

Abbreviations .... **iv**
Preface .... **v**
1. Basic data and background **1**
2. Mortality data **2**
   2.1. Geographical variation in child mortality 3
   2.2. Cause-specific mortality 5
   2.3. Demographic and socioeconomic determinants
         of child mortality 6
3. Progress towards achieving MDG 4 .... **9**
   3.1. Summary of progress 9
   3.2. Interventions 9
   3.3. Monitoring progress towards targets 12
   3.4. Health care delivery strategies 13
4. Health system **14**
   4.1 Policies, strategies and legislation 14
   4.2 Human resources 16
   4.3 Collection of evidence and information
         for policy-making and planning 21
   4.4 Child health financing 21
5. Collaboration and coordination **26**
References **28**

Abbreviations

ARI	Acute Respiratory Infection
CDHS	Cambodia Demographic and Health Survey
CIPS	Cambodia Inter-Censal Population Survey
CMDGs	Cambodia Millennium Development Goals
CNCC	Cambodian National Council for Children
CRC	Convention on the Rights of the Child
CPA	Comprehensive Package of Activities
EU	European Union
HIV/AIDS	Human Immunodeficiency Virus / Acquired Immunodeficiency Syndrome
IMCI	Integrated Management of Childhood Illness
IMR	Infant Mortality Rate
GAVI	Global Alliance for Vaccines and Immunization
GDP	Gross Domestic Product
GFATM	Global Fund to Fight HIV/AIDS, Tuberculosis and Malaria
MCH	Maternal and Child Health
MPA	Minimum Package of Activities
NGO	Nongovernmental Organization
NMR	Neonatal Mortality Rate
ORS	Oral Rehydration Salts
ORT	Oral Rehydration Therapy
PNMR	Post-neonatal Mortality Rate
STI	Sexually Transmitted Infection
U5MR	Under-five Mortality Rate
UNICEF	United Nations Children's Fund
USAID	United States Agency for International Development
WFDP	Workforce Development Plan
WHO	World Health Organization

Preface

Approximately 3000 children under five years of age die every day in the Western Pacific Region from common preventable and treatable conditions including diarrhoea, pneumonia and perinatal events. Many of these deaths are associated with undernutrition. Vaccine preventable diseases and injuries further contribute to this high number of childhood deaths.

The Millennium Development Goal 4 of the United Nations Millennium Declaration calls for a reduction by two thirds, between 1990 and 2015, of the under-five mortality rate. An analysis of the progress in the Region shows that the achievement of the goal will prove challenging for many countries if mortality reduction continues to stagnate and preventable and treatable causes of childhood mortality persist.

The WHO/UNICEF Regional Child Survival Strategy outlines a unified direction to accelerate and sustain action towards achieving the national targets for Millennium Development Goal 4, and to reduce inequities in child survival, particularly in areas of greatest need. The strategy was endorsed by the WHO Regional Committee for the Western Pacific at its fifty-sixth session in September 2005.

The Strategy focuses on the implementation of an Essential Package for Child Survival composed of seven intervention areas: (1) skilled attendance during pregnancy, delivery and the immediate postpartum period; (2) care of the newborn; (3) breastfeeding and complementary feeding; (4) micronutrient supplementation; (5) immunization of children and mothers; (6) integrated management of sick children; and (7) the use of insecticide-treated bednets in areas where malaria is a problem. At the heart of the Strategy are 10 core child survival indicators for the monitoring of progress towards universal coverage of the different intervention areas.

The Western Pacific Region is a very diverse area. Therefore, the successful implementation of child survival actions at the country level must first take into account the local child health situation and health system capacity. The child survival country profiles have been developed with support from WHO in collaboration with the respective Ministries of Health. Each profile includes information on the progress towards implementation of Millennium Development Goal 4, the current status of the evidence-based interventions that affect the survival of children, related policies and strategies, child health financing, and coordination mechanisms.

This compilation should be useful in further analysing and designing country-specific plans of action, coordinating activities with key stakeholders, and tracking progress towards the universal coverage of essential child survival interventions. These profiles reflect the current picture of child survival. Once new data become available, and further progress in child survival intervention coverage is noted, these profiles may need to be updated.

1. Basic data and background

Cambodia has a population of 13.09 million,[1] with 11.1%, or 1.45 million children under five years of age (sex ratio 1:1). The birth registration rate was 66.4% in 2005.[2] Adult literacy stands at 73.6%: 64.1% for females and 84.7% for males.[3] Other key background information relevant to child survival is summarized in Table 1.

Table 1: Country background statistics

Population (million)	[Total]		13.09 (2004)	Life expectancy at birth (years)[4]	[Male]	58.57 (2006)
	[0-4 years]	11.1%	1.45 (2004)		[Female]	64.85 (2006)
	[5-14 years]	27.5%	3.60 (2004)			
	[15-19 years]	11.7%	1.53 (2004)	Birth registration[2]		66.4% (2005)
Annual population growth rate			1.81% (2004)	Total fertility rate[2]		3.4 (2005)
Under-five mortality rate[2] (per 1 000 live births)			83 (2005)	Percentage of population served with safe water[1]	[Total]	44% (2004)
					[Urban]	72% (2004)
					[Rural]	40% (2004)
Infant mortality rate[2] (per 1 000 live births)			66 (2005)	Percentage of population with adequate sanitary facilities	[Total]	21% (2000)
					[Urban]	60% (2000)
					[Rural]	14% (2000)
Maternal mortality rate[2] (per 100 000 live births)			472 (2005)	GDP per capita (USD)[5]		419 (2006)
				Human Development Index and Rank[6]	0.583 (2006)	129 (2006)

Source: Country Health Information Profiles WHO, 2006 unless specifically referenced.

After decades of war and civil strife, Cambodia is developing economically and socially but remains one of the poorest countries in Asia. The latest socio-economic household survey in 2004 found that 35% of Cambodians live below the national poverty line, compared to 47% in 1993/94 surveys.[7] Even the poor have experienced an improvement in living standards but inequity is significantly increasing in health and education. Poverty in Cambodia predominantly affects rural households and is associated with landlessness, remoteness from markets and services, lack of productive assets, low levels of education and high dependency ratios. Poor people are more vulnerable to ill health and high out-of-pocket health payments are a major cause of debt and loss of land.[8]

2. Mortality data

Population-based data on early childhood mortality rates are collected through large-scale surveys. The latest most reliable source with a nationally representative sample is the Report of Cambodia Demographic and Health Survey (CDHS) 2005.[2] Based on the trends identified in the Inter-Censal Population Survey in 2004 and CDHS 2005, Cambodia showed a substantial decline in early child mortality rates since 2000 (see Table 2).

Table 2: Early childhood mortality rates expressed per 1000 live births, 2000 and 2005

Year	Neonatal mortality (NM)	Post-neonatal mortality (PNM)	Infant mortality	Child mortality	Under-five mortality
2000	37	58	95	33	124
2005	28	37	66	19	83
2005 (% of U5M)	34%	46%	80%	23%	
2005 (% of Infant mortality)	42%	56%			

Source: Cambodia Demographic and Health Survey 2000, 2005.

2.1. Geographical variation in child mortality

Figures 1 and 2 show the regional variations in under-five and infant mortality rates.[2] The highest rates were found in the remote and scarcely populated provinces of the North-East, and in the densely populated agricultural provinces of the central plains.

Figure 1: Under-five mortality rates per 1000 live births, by province

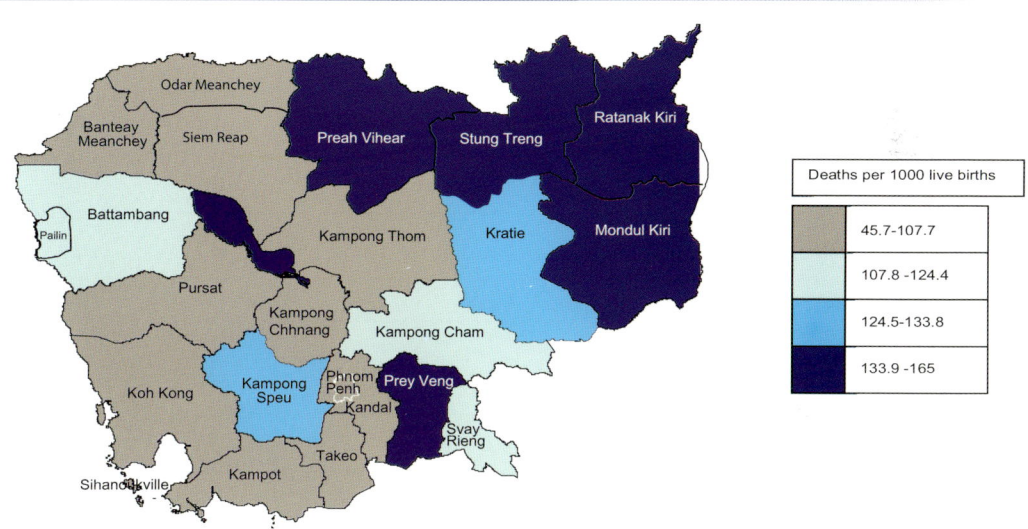

Source: Cambodia Demographic and Health Survey 2005.

Figure 2: Infant mortality rates per 1000 live births, by province

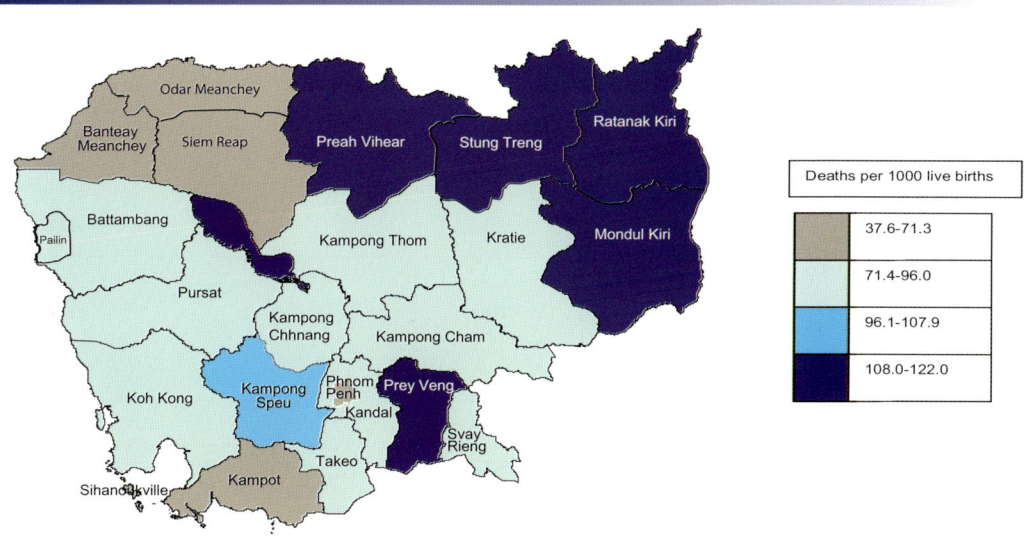

Source: Cambodia Demographic and Health Survey 2005.

Table 3: Early childhood mortality rates (per 1000 live births)

Provinces (Clusters)	Neonatal mortality (0-28 days)	Post-neonatal mortality (1-11 mo)	Infant mortality (<12 mo)	Child mortality (12-59 mo)	Under-five mortality (< 60 mo)
Kampong Cham	35	60	94	18	111
Battambang/Krong Pailin	29	68	97	21	116
Kandal	30	55	85	18	101
Prey Veng	52	69	121	25	143
Kampong Chhnang	36	51	87	15	101
Takeo	52	43	96	7	102
Kampot/Krong Kep/ Krong Preah Sihanouk	37	30	67	17	83
Pursat	27	59	86	21	106
Banteay Meanchey	34	42	76	22	96
Kampong Speu	41	66	107	17	122
Siem Reap/ Odar Meanchey	34	33	67	29	94
Preah Vihear/ Stung Treng	34	77	111	39	146
Kratie	37	47	84	34	116
Svay Rieng	29	64	92	20	110
Mondul Kiri/ Ratanak Kiri	56	65	122	50	165
Kampong Thom	38	49	87	20	106
Phnom Penh	24	18	42	10	52
Koh Kong	37	50	88	18	104
National	**28**	**37**	**66**	**19**	**83**

Source: Cambodia Demographic and Health Survey 2005.

2.2. Cause-specific mortality

Population-based data on causes of death are not available. The National Health Statistics of the Ministry of Health provides data for public health facilities. WHO has provided estimates applicable to high child mortality countries in the Western Pacific Region, as shown in Figures 3a and 3b. According to these estimates, the leading direct causes of early childhood deaths are acute respiratory infections (mainly pneumonia), diarrhoeal diseases and neonatal conditions. Malaria, dengue fever and HIV/AIDS do not result in a considerable burden of child mortality. Figure 3c shows the causes of under-five mortality at hospital level.

Figure 3: Causes of under-five and neonatal mortality in Cambodia

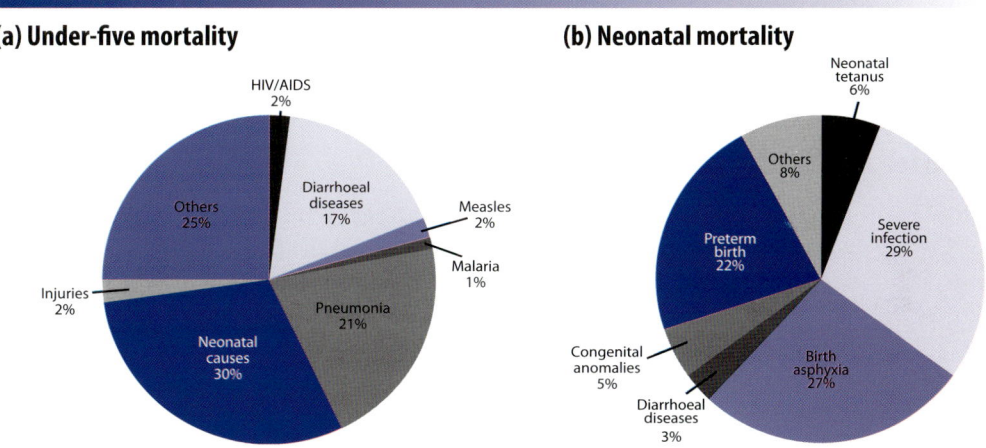

Source: Annual estimated proportion of deaths by cause for children, 2000. World Health Organization.

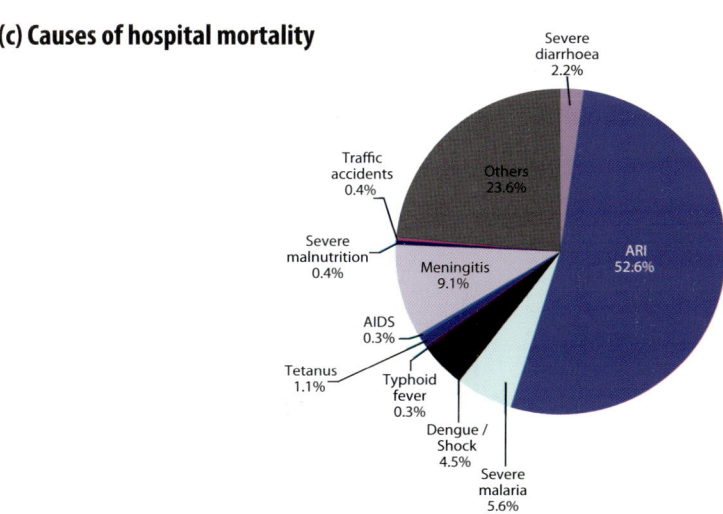

Source: National Health Statistics, 2006.

Estimates of possible cause-specific mortality from verbal autopsy data from the CDHS 2005 show congruence with the WHO estimates, that respiratory infection remains the leading cause of death amongst post-neonatal infants and young children (30%), followed by diarrhoea (27%), dengue hemorrhagic fever (11%), severe acute undernutrition (7.5%) and measles (6.5%). Although the under-five and infant mortality rates have decreased significantly, the neonatal mortality rate has only slightly decreased. Twenty-five percent of these neonates are of low birth weight and about 20% had a difficult delivery. A quarter had a history of poor feeding after initially feeding well, indicating possible sepsis, with 7% also having convulsions indicating neonatal tetanus. Greater efforts to focus on reducing neonatal deaths need to be taken. National data from the CDHS reveal that 80% of under-five deaths occur in the first year of life, 46% during the post-neonatal period and 34% during the neonatal period.

2.3. Demographic and socioeconomic determinants of child mortality

The chances of child survival depend on whether a child comes from a poor or better-off household, the level of mother's education and residency in an urban or rural area (see Figures 4a and 4b). The CDHS 2005 shows that the mortality rate gap between the rich and poor has widened in the last five years (see Figure 4c).

Figure 4a: Early childhood mortality in rural and urban areas

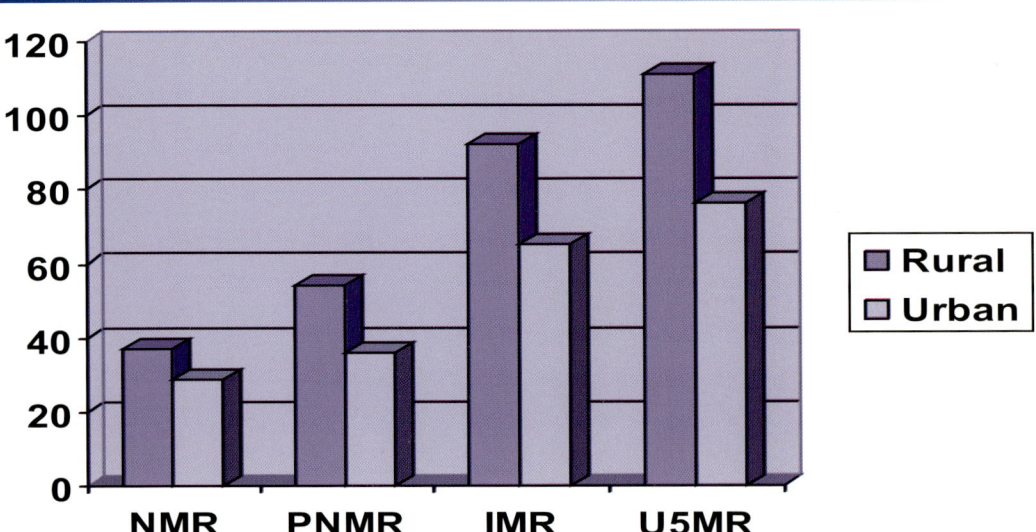

Source: Cambodia Demographic and Health Survey 2005.

Figure 4b: Early childhood mortality by family income and mother's education

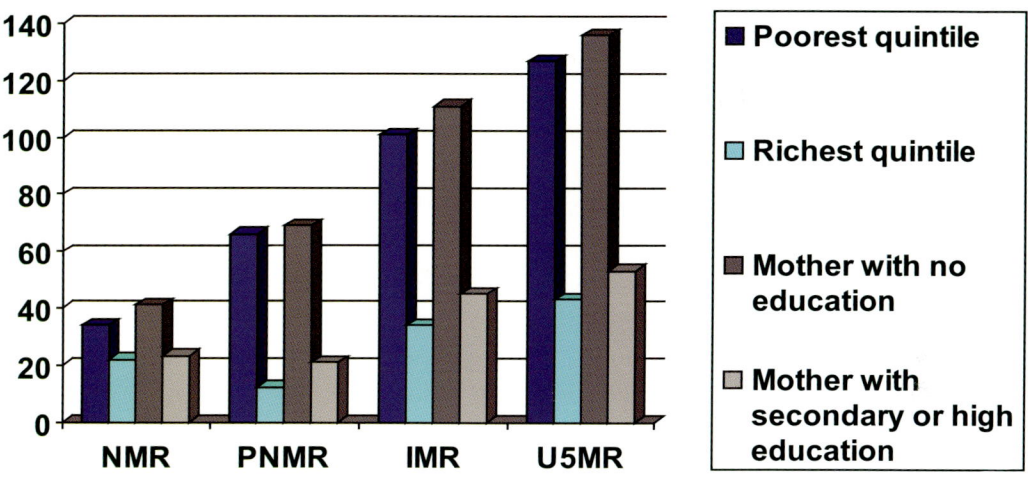

Source: Cambodia Demographic and Health Survey 2005.

Figure 4c: Early childhood mortality by health quintiles, 2000 and 2005

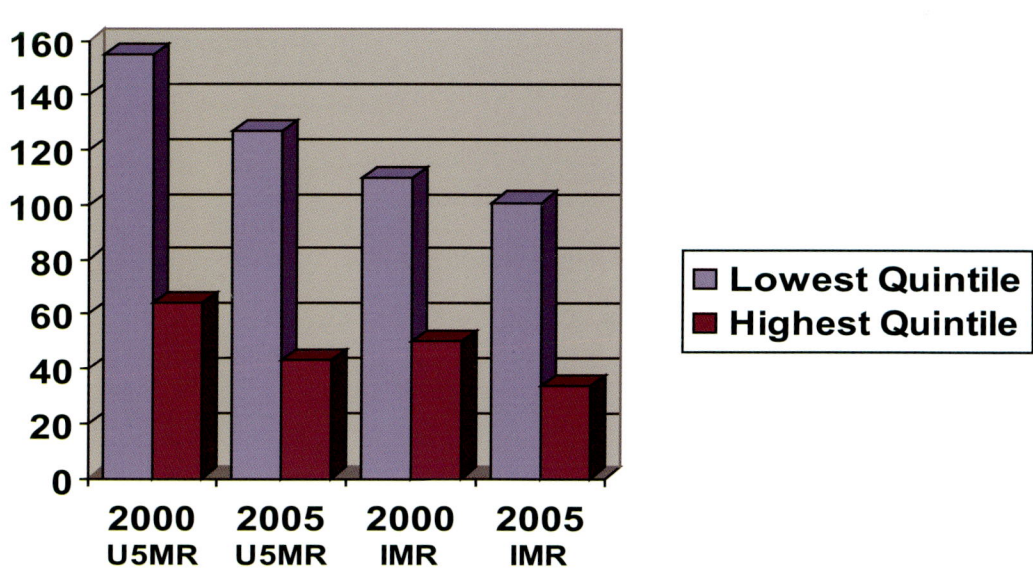

Source: Cambodia Demographic and Health Survey, 2000, 2005.

From 1990 to 2003, there was limited reduction in child mortality as summarized in the Benchmark Report,[10] which came to the following conclusions:

- After a steep decline in the 1980s in early childhood mortality rates, this trend has slowed down considerably in the 1990s (see Figure 5). Two-thirds of childhood deaths occur in the post-neonatal period, with some indication of an increased mortality rate in this age group.
- By 2000, there had been little progress in the major risk factors for child mortality. High undernutrition rates prevailed, access to and utilization of health services lingered at low levels, as did access to safe drinking water and sanitation. Low female literacy rate persisted.

However, by 2005, there were significant reductions in child mortality rates (see Figure 5).

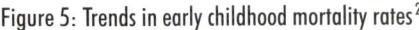

Figure 5: Trends in early childhood mortality rates[2]

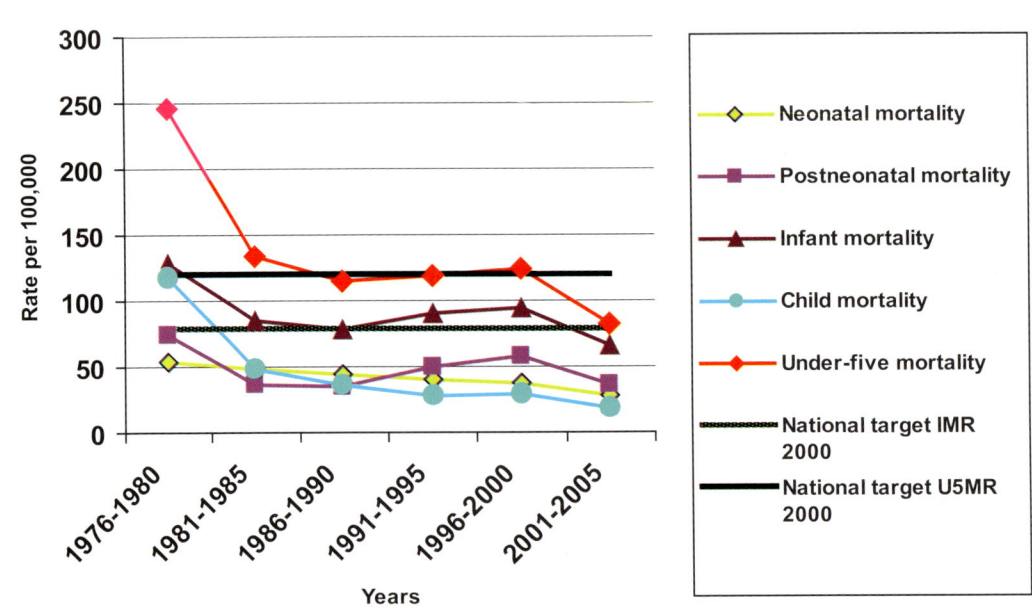

3. Progress towards achieving MDG 4

3.1. Summary of progress

In 2003, the Government issued the *Cambodia Millennium Development Goals Report*, outlining the country-specific Cambodia Millennium Development Goals (CMDGs) to be reached by 2015.[11] Key targets of the CMDGs include reduction of the under-five and infant mortality rates. Following the country's commitment to the Millennium Development Goals (MDGs), the Government and development partners are harmonizing their planning and programming around the CMDGs, which form the bases of the National Strategic Development Plan 2006-2010.[12]

Table 4. Progress towards achieving MDG 4

Indicator	2000 (CDHS)	2005 (CDHS)	Target for 2015
Under-five mortality rate (per 1000 live births)	124	83	65
Infant mortality rate (per 1000 live births)	95	66	50
Proportion of one-year-old children immunized against measles	41%	70%	90%

The CDHS 2005 indicates that Cambodia is now back on track to achieving the CMDGs. The Ministry of Health has made maternal and child health a top priority for the coming years in order to achieve these targets.

3.2. Interventions

In mid-2004, responding to the slow progress towards MDG 4, the Child Survival Partnership High Level Consultation on Millennium Development Goal 4 "Reducing Child Mortality in Cambodia", was convened in Phnom Penh. Prior to this, successful national programmes aimed at delivering health interventions to reduce child mortality had included the National Immunization Programme, which made possible poliomyelitis elimination and the considerable drop in measles cases starting in 2000; the National Vitamin A Programme which increased vitamin A supplementation coverage; the National Dengue Programme which had reduced hospital mortality through improved case management; and the programme for the control of HIV/AIDS, which had been expanded. These programmes had four elements of success: clear targets, strong commitment from the Government and donors, clear definitions of responsibilities, and sufficient funding. Coverage of preventive measures such as vitamin A supplementation and deworming have increased. However, health interventions addressing the main killers of children: pneumonia, diarrhoea, neonatal causes and undernutrition were not given sufficient attention or resources, particularly in rural and remote areas.

By 2005, the health sector reform process showed some progress in effectively delivering the minimum and comprehensive packages of activities which included preventive and curative interventions. However, access was not entirely equitable across different wealth quintiles (see Figure 6).

Figure 6: Disparities in health service delivery and nutrition indicators by wealth ranking
(Note: trained personnel include doctors, nurses and midwives)

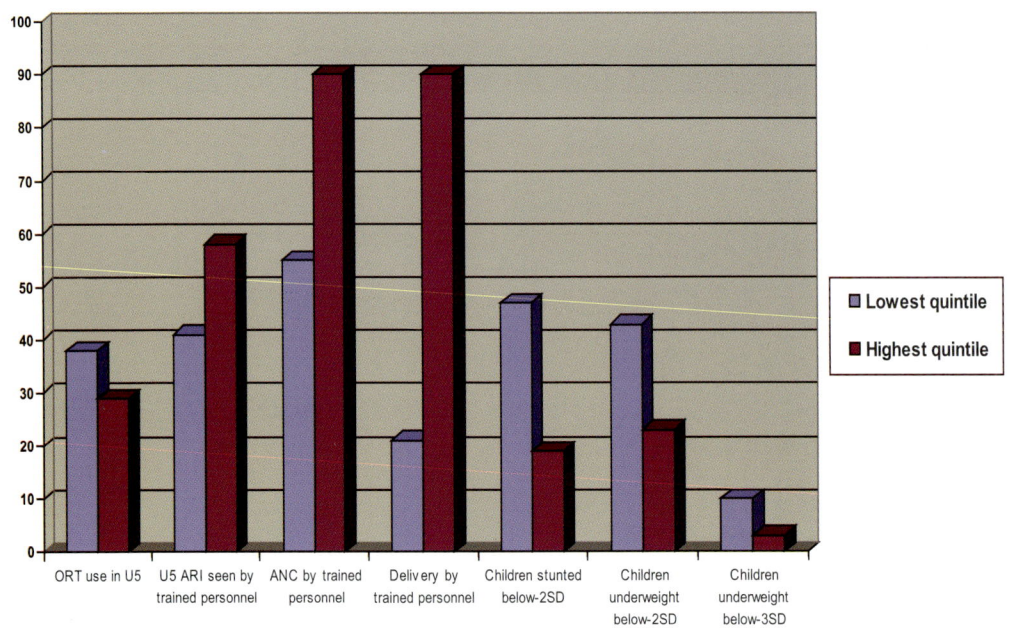

Source: Cambodia Demographic and Health Survey 2005.

To reduce child mortality in Cambodia, the Child Survival Partnership High Level Consultation on Millennium Development Goal 4 and the subsequent National Child Survival Conference and nongovernmental organization consultation workshop, endorsed selected high-impact child survival interventions summarized in the Cambodia Child Survival Score Card, together with clear targets for 2007 and updated targets for 2010 (see Table 5).

Table 5. The Cambodia child survival score card

Intervention	CDHS 2000	CDHS 2005	Target 2007[1]	Target 2010	Universal Coverage
Early initiation of breastfeeding	11%	35%	35%	60%	99%
Exclusive breastfeeding	11%	60%	25%	80%	90%
Complementary feeding	71%	82%	95%	95%	99%
Vitamin A	29%	35%	80%	85%	99%
Measles vaccine	55%	77%	80%	92%	99%
Tetanus toxoid	30%	54%	70%	80%	99%
Insecticide treated nets (ITNs)	9% (3-38%)[2]	4.2% (11-37%)[3]	80%	80%	99%
Vector control (*Aedes aegypti*)[4]	181 Sites	-	<10 Sites	<10 Sites	<10 Sites
Oral rehydration therapy (ORT)	74%	58%	80%	85%	99%
Antibiotic for pneumonia	35%	48%[5]	50%	75%	99%
Malaria treatment	-	(0.3-3.3%)[6]	85%	95%	99%
Skilled birth attendance	32%	44%	60%	70%	99%

[1] NOTE: These targets were set for the 2003-2007 Health Sector Strategic Plan.
[2] 9% is the national average; in the provinces with high malaria transmission (Koh Kong, Kratie, Mondul Kiri, Preah Vihear, Ratana Kiri and Stung Traeng) insecticide-treated net coverage ranged from 3 to 38%.
[3] 4.2% is the national average; in the provinces with high malaria transmission – Preah Vihear/Stoung Treng, Mondul Kiri/Ratana Kiri,Odar Meanchey, Kratie, Koh Kong – the use varied from 11-37%.
[4] Given the increasing contribution of dengue fever to under-five mortality in Cambodia the Child Survival Steering Committee has decided to include vector control in the Scorecard; vector control for *Aedes aegypti* is the most important public health intervention to prevent dengue fever. The indicator used is the Breteau Index defined as: number of positive breeding sites per 100 houses (%) surveyed. Effective vector control is achieved when there are less than 10 breeding sites per 100 houses surveyed (<10%).
[5] 48% represent a proportion of children under 5 with signs of ARI (cough and fast breathing) taken to a health facility or provider.
[6] In Preah Vihear/Stoung Treng, Mondul Kiri/Ratana Kiri, Odar Meanchey, Kratie, Koh Kong – the proportion of children who received anti-malarial treatment varied from 0.3-3.3%.

Eleven of the 23 child survival interventions that have been identified as most cost-effective and evidence-based[13] are included in the Cambodia Child Survival Score Card. Some interventions, including access to safe water, sanitation and hygiene, are subsumed under broader strategic approaches. Other interventions, such as antibiotics for dysentery, zinc treatment for diarrhoea, vitamin A treatment for measles and severe undernutrition, and newborn health interventions, except antenatal steroids, are included in either Integrated Management of Childhood Illness (IMCI) or Safe Motherhood assessment and management protocols. In addition, dengue prevention (by vector control) is also included in the Cambodia score card interventions as dengue haemorrhagic fever is rapidly becoming a large contributor to child mortality in Cambodia. However, there are a few interventions that have been excluded for the time being, for reasons that will be discussed briefly below:

- Zinc supplementation – Zinc tablets are now on the essential drug list for treatment of diarrhoea (10-day course) but there is no current recommendation for daily zinc supplementation in Cambodia.
- Hib vaccine, Rotavirus vaccine, Pneumococcal conjugate vaccine – These vaccines are not included in current immunization guidelines in Cambodia.
- Japanese Encephalitis vaccine - A disease burden surveillance study is ongoing.
- Antimalarial intermittent preventive treatment in pregnancy – This is currently being reviewed for areas with high malaria prevalence.
- Antenatal steroids – This is relevant only for hospital deliveries.
- Antiretroviral treatment and replacement feeding in the HIV context– Preventive treatment with zidovudine or zidovudine and nevirapine is currently recommended for HIV-positive mothers. Replacement feeding is not provided and hence not generally recommended. Mothers are encouraged to make informed choices on infant feeding after counseling. Replacement feeding is only recommended if it is acceptable, feasible, affordable, sustainable and safe.[14]

3.3. Monitoring progress towards targets

Progress towards targets is being monitored through joint annual performance reviews of the health sector using the score card indicators, which are collected regularly through national health statistics and surveys. Despite a generally positive tendency, overall progress has been uneven, with those interventions more dependent on curative services and functional health facilities lagging behind. Ongoing monitoring for national health statistics needs to be strengthened at provincial, operational district and health centre levels. Some interventions will require population-based surveys for monitoring (e.g. rate of exclusive breastfeeding). These surveys may also be useful to get a more complete picture of intervention coverage as the national health statistics may not cover the private sector.

3.4. Health care delivery strategies

The main delivery strategies for achieving universal coverage of the selected essential child survival interventions include integrated outreach, the health centre-based delivery of the minimum package of activities (MPA), and the comprehensive package of activities (CPA) for referral hospitals. There are also other delivery strategies for the same interventions that are not currently applied to their full potential or address specific circumstances only. These include social marketing of ORS and early differential diagnosis and treatment of malaria, acute respiratory infections and childhood diarrhoea in remote communities by village malaria workers. The responsibility for reaching universal coverage is shared between vertical programmes and local health authorities, as illustrated in the matrix (see Figure 7). The matrix is also a useful tool to monitor progress towards universal coverage of all essential child survival interventions.

Figure 7. Child survival implementation matrix

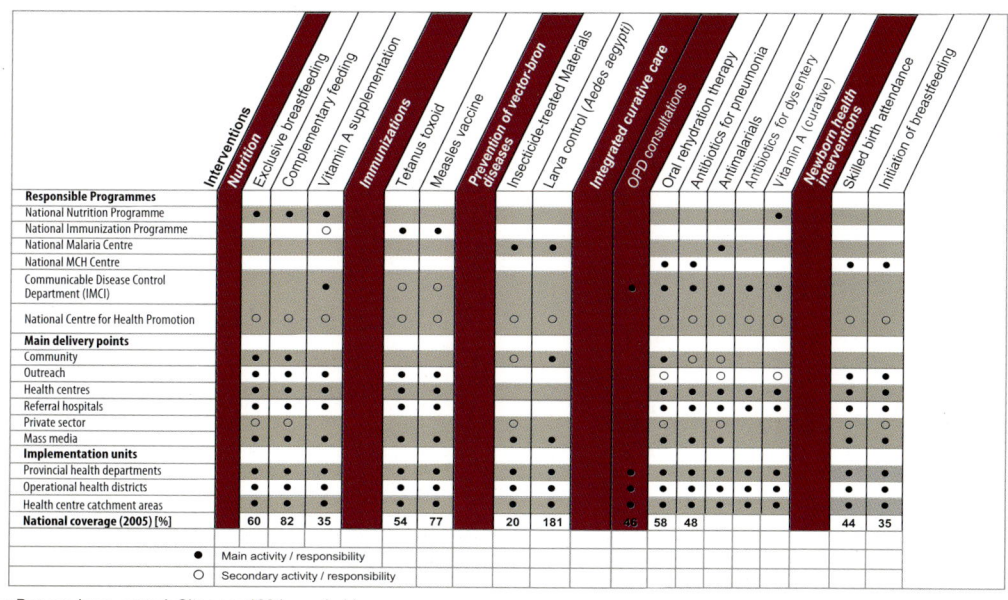

Note: Dengue larva control: Sites per 100 households.

4. Health system

In the 1990s, the Government introduced health system reforms to improve and extend primary health care through the implementation of a district health system focusing on the distribution of facilities in accordance with a health coverage plan and the allocation of financial resources to provinces. Operational districts are composed of 100 000 to 200 000 people, with a referral hospital providing a comprehensive package of activities and health centres delivering primary health care to a target population of 10 000 through a minimum package of activities.

4.1. Policies, strategies and legislation

There are a number of legal provisions, policies and strategies that relate directly to child survival. These are summarized in Table 6.

Table 6. Legislation, policies and strategies related to child survival

Description	Topic	Content
Legislation		
Constitution	Commitment to United Nations Human Rights Conventions	"The Kingdom of Cambodia shall recognise and respect human rights as stipulated in the United Nations Charter, the Universal Declaration of Human Rights, the covenants and conventions related to human rights, women's and children's rights" (Article 31)
	Right to life and protection	"The State shall protect the rights of children, as stipulated in the Convention on Children, in particular, the right to life...[and]... protect children from acts that are injurious to their education opportunities, health and welfare." (Article 48)
	Right to health care	"The health of the people shall be guaranteed. The State shall give full consideration to disease prevention and medical treatment. Poor citizens shall receive free medical consultation in public hospitals, infirmaries and maternities." (Article 72) "The State shall give full consideration to children and mothers..." (Article 73)

Table 6. Legislation, policies and strategies related to child survival (Continued)

Description	Topic	Content
Labour Act of 1992	Child labour (up to 18 years)	Health protection for children (below 18 yrs) working in factories
Sub-decree on Marketing of Products for Infant and Young Child Feeding (2005) Joint Circular for the Implementation of the sub-decree 2006-2007	Marketing of breast-milk substitutes	Protection from harmful marketing practices
Health Financing Charter (1996)	Cost recovery	Legal basis for charging patients fees for services provided by public facilities
Policies and strategies		
Guidelines for Developing Operational Districts [1997]	Functioning of operational health districts	Managerial guidelines for district managers
National Vitamin A Policy Guidelines [2000] Updated in 2001, 2007	Vitamin A supplementation	Policy statement for vitamin A capsule supplementation for children aged 6-59 months and women with eight weeks postpartum, together with implementation guidelines
National Policy on Infant and Young Child Feeding [2000]		Official feeding recommendations for children aged 0-24 months
IMCI Case Management Guidelines and Feeding Recommendations defining the minimum package of activities (MPA 10) [2002] Updated in 2006	Integrated case management of the sick child	Clinical case management guidelines for sick children for the minimum package of activities, with feeding recommendations
National Treatment Guidelines for Malaria [2004]	Malaria treatment	Clinical treatment guidelines recommending artemisinine-based combination therapy
National Policy Prevention of Mother-Child Transmission of HIV [2005]	Prevention of mother-to-child HIV transmission	Prevention of mother-to-child transmission of HIV
Strategic Plan for Reproductive Health in Cambodia [2006-2010]	Reproductive health	Includes maternal and newborn health, adolescent reproductive and sexual health, STI/HIV/AIDS, birth spacing and gender equality
Cambodia Child Survival Startegy [2006]	Child survival	Outlines the approach to reducing child mortality in Cambodia and achieving the Cambodia Millennium Development Goal 4

The Health Sector Strategic Plan 2003-2007 lays out seven goals for the health system of which four are related to child survival: reduced infant mortality rate, reduced child mortality rate, improved nutritional status among children and women, and reduced total fertility rate. These goals are to be achieved through a focus on key areas of health service delivery, behavioural change, quality improvement, human resource development, health financing and institutional development.[15] A new Health Sector Strategic Plan for 2008-2015 is being developed with expected emphasis on maternal, newborn and child health.

All five priorities set by the Ministry of Health for 2005-2006 at the 2005 Ministry of Health Joint Annual Performance Review directly address key areas: emergency obstetric care, skilled birth attendance, IMCI, birth spacing services, enabling health centres to deliver a full minimum package of activities. These were further endorsed as top priorities of the Ministry of Health at the 2007 Joint Annual Performance Review together with the full implementation of the Child Survival Scorecard Interventions.

The Kingdom of Cambodia assented to the Convention on the Rights of the Child (CRC) on 15 October 1992.

4.2. Human resources

The health sector reform process also included substantial work on rebuilding human resources for health. In 1996, the Ministry of Health produced its first Work Force Development Plan (WFDP) for 1996-2005 and currently a new plan for 2006-2015 is under development. The WFDP 1996-2005 identified the main categories of health personnel employed in government health services, set out the cadre of health workers and the training requirement for each cadre, and predicted training and recruitment needs for the future (see Table 7).

Table 7. Human resources for health by main categories in the public health sector (excluding armed forces)

Category	Numbers	Description
Nursing personnel	7901	There are two categories of nurses, secondary and primary. Secondary nurses train for three years, primary for one year.
Primary nurses	(3335)	Primary nurse training has ceased.
Secondary nurses	(4566)	The Nursing Education Programme is now a three-year diploma course and includes basic midwifery and training.
		There is a two-year post graduate anaesthesia nurse training programme.

Table 7. Human resources for health by main categories in the public health sector (excluding armed forces) (Continued)

Category	Numbers	Description
Midwives	2850	The current midwifery training has changed to a four-year training programme that includes the three-year nursing diploma and one year of post-basic specialist training in advanced midwifery and child health. Previously there were programmes for primary midwives (one-year course) and secondary midwives (three-year course), with direct registration after school.
Primary midwives	(1076)	A one-year direct entry midwifery course was restarted in the North East region.
Secondary midwives	(1774)	
Medical assistants	1317	Medical assistants undertook a five-year pre-service education at the Faculty of Medicine. This course was last offered in 1994.
Medical doctors	2079	Medical doctors undertake a seven-year pre-service education at the Faculty of Medicine and one year of supervised public service in the health sector to become fully qualified.
Medical specialists		In 1997, three-year specialist-training programmes in internal medicine, surgery, paediatrics, obstetrics and gynaecology and pathology were introduced. Ten paediatricians were trained. The WFDP identified the need for a minimum of 30 paediatric specialists for a population of 10 million.
Dental health personnel	242	Dental personnel include dentists, dental assistants and dental nurses. Dental nurses provide chairside assistance only.
Dentists	(137)	Dentists undertake a seven-year education at the Faculty of Medicine.
Dental assistants	(83)	Dental assistants' training stopped in 1994. Dental assistants undertake a five-year education and dental nurses a six-month training course.
Primary dentists	(22)	

Table 7. Human resources for health by main categories in the public health sector (excluding armed forces) (Continued)

Category	Numbers	Description
Pharmacy personnel	557	Pharmacy personnel include doctors involved in pharmacy, pharmacists and pharmacy assistants.
Pharmacists	(377)	A doctor in pharmacy is required to complete at least four years of postgraduate training and a pharmacist five years of training at the School of Pharmacy in the Faculty of Medicine.
Pharmacy assistants	(143)	Pharmacist assistant training stopped in 1994. Pharmacy assistants completed a four-year course.
Others	not available	Other cadres of health staff include primary and secondary laboratory technicians with training lasting three years and one year, respectively, physiotherapists (three years of training), health agents (who trained for one year during the Khmer Rouge period on environmental health issues).
Informal health care providers	not available	A number of informal health care providers have been involved in promoting health, but also in the provision of certain services and commodities. These include traditional birth attendants, community health volunteers, drugsellers, community-based distributors of contraceptives, and village malaria workers. No standardized training exists for these categories and none of these approaches are implemented nationwide. A large number of informal short training courses exist.

Source: National Health Statistics 2005.

Between 1996 and 2003, the ratio of secondary to primary nurses and midwives changed and there were some improvements in the distribution of staff (see Figure 8). The number of secondary nurses and midwives employed in areas outside Phnom Penh increased and the number employed in Phnom Penh decreased (see Table 8).

Table 8. Changes in the nursing / midwifery workforce 1996 - 2005

	Nurses						Midwives					
	1996		2003		2005		1996		2003		2005	
	Secondary nurse	Primary nurse	Secondary nurse	Primary nurse	Secondary nurse	Primary nurse	Secondary midwife	Primary midwife	Secondary midwife	Primary midwife	Secondary midwife	Primary midwife
Phnom Penh	1357	337	1278	250	1114	140	419	52	372	42	267	10
Rest of Cambodia	2622	4093	3266	3174	3452	3195	1287	1463	1445	1061	1507	1066
Total	3979	4430	4544	3424	4566	3335	1706	1515	1817	1103	1774	1076

The termination of primary-nurse and all direct-entry midwifery training has resulted in a 10% decrease in the number of midwives and a 5% decrease in the number of nurses in the Ministry of Health workforce since 1996. In 2005, there were 224 health centres without a midwife at all. While there has been an increase in the intake of nursing and post-graduate midwifery courses, the output is still short of the required staff numbers needed to provide safe coverage in public health facilities.[16]

Figure 8: Growth of health workforce in Cambodia, 1996 - 2005

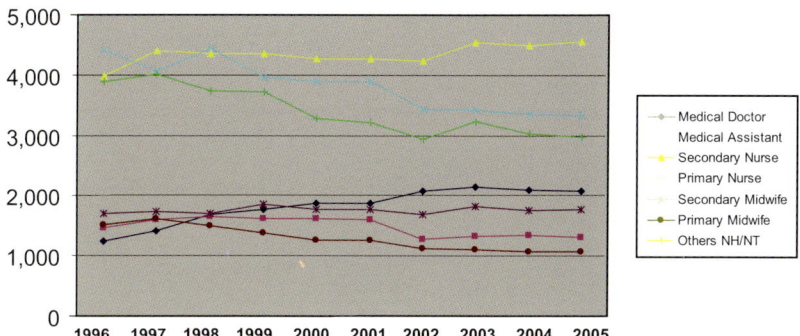

To date, the overall ratio of Ministry of Health physicians (comprised of medical doctors and medical assistants) to population is approximately 1:5200. The ratio of nurses is 1:2616 and midwives 1:6229. There is a marked disparity between Ministry of Health workers in Phnom Penh and the rest of Cambodia. Phnom Penh has 9.3% of the population and 25.1% of all Ministry staff. The north-east provinces have 3.7% of the population and 5.6% of the Ministry of Health staff, and the rest of Cambodia has 87% of the population and 69.4% of the Ministry staff.

There have been difficulties in posting staff to rural areas for economic and social reasons, resulting in mal-distribution of the workforce. The concentration of specialists in Phnom Penh especially in national hospitals and Ministry of Health Central Office obscures the real shortages in the provinces. Only 51% of doctors, 54% of pharmacists, 57% of physiotherapists, and 57% of x-ray specialists are distributed in the 24 provinces.[16] Some effort has been made to realistically assess recruitment needs, target priority cadres (midwives) for recruitment and appoint staff to vacant posts, but more work is needed to ensure that personnel actually work in the posts to which they are assigned.

The Benchmark Report[10] concluded that, in order to improve child survival, human resources have to be able to deliver the essential interventions in a more efficient and skilful manner. To improve the delivery of maternal and newborn care interventions, as well as curative and nutrition interventions, it is necessary to fulfill the following three pre-conditions: health centres must have staff with updated midwifery skills, IMCI should be implemented, and the key nutrition interventions included in the minimum package of activities should be delivered. Since 2000, considerable progress has been made towards fulfilling these three pre-conditions. Efforts to train and deploy trained midwives to all health centres have been going on for some time, while IMCI implementation at the district level only started in 2001, and training of health centre staff in the nutrition component of the minimum package of activities (MPA 10) only began in 2004 (see Figure 9).

Figure 9: Coverage of child health survival packages

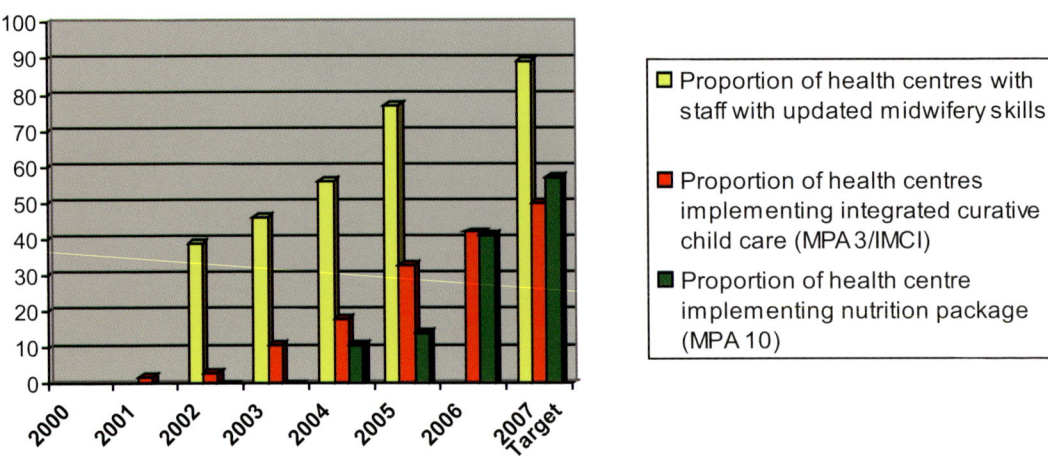

A priority plan for training was developed in 2000, based on the agreed need to upgrade the knowledge and skills of the existing workforce. Priority for training was given to upgrading the skills of current Ministry of Health staff through in-service training using modules on the MPA and CPA service packages. MPA/CPA modules are currently being updated. The Midwifery Review (2006) highlighted the need for strengthening pre-service training of midwives for both knowledge and skills.[17]

In 2004, 43% of health centres were with staff without updated midwifery skills. To overcome this shortage, a one-year midwifery training programme was reintroduced in the north-east provinces in 2003. By 2005, there was improvement with only 24% of health centres having staff without updated midwifery skills, although the Midwifery Review indicated that their skills were still inadequate. [17]

In most training programmes, the clinical experience for trainees is inadequate. A formal process for the recognition of training hospitals is now being established. There are no systems in place to ensure the quality of graduates through registration or licensing. The advent of a number of private training institutes in the past few years makes the introduction of some form of quality assurance for health-worker training imperative.

Besides qualifications, skills and deployment problems across the country, the main human resource challenge remains to be the persistently low salaries in the public health system, resulting in low staff motivation, absenteeism and widespread 'under-the-table' payments. Although different remedial or coping mechanisms, including contracting out of services, user fees, granting of per diems for specific activities and provision of training have been used as incentives, a comprehensive and sustainable solution to the problem is still lacking.

4.3. Collection of evidence and information for policy-making and planning

Collection of evidence and information for policy decisions and planning remains a challenge. Vital registration is not yet reliable. The national health information system only covers public health facilities, representing only a small share of all health services provided in the country. The quality of data is still to be improved. Information from private providers has been collected only recently for a very limited range of health topics and with limited coverage. Large-scale population-based surveys (e.g. Cambodia Demographic and Health Survey; Cambodia Inter-Censal Population Survey; Cambodia Socio-Economic Survey) collecting health indicators are carried out every three to five years, not always with comparable methodologies and indicators. Smaller scale population-based surveys, often carried out by NGOs, are not systematically compiled and also follow variable methodologies. In particular, information on causes of death and epidemiology is lacking. The most reliable sources of information on the child survival score card indicators are the Demographic and Health Surveys and a very limited number of other surveys. Information on financial resource allocation is also patchy and incomplete.

4.4. Child health financing

Government health expenditure has been increasing. In 1999, the total recurrent government expenditure on health was US$ 2.85 per capita; in 2005, it was US$ 4 per capita. Overall health sector financing in Cambodia absorbs 12%–13% of GDP, which is the highest among developing countries in Asia. Its three main financing sources are private, mainly out-of-pocket payments, donors and government revenues. An estimated 70% is from out-of-pocket payments, representing approximately US$ 24.00 per capita. Overall, however, health care costs have dropped considerably in both the private and public sectors in the last five years as evidenced by data from the CDHS 2005. Although government health expenditure has been increasing in recent years, donors are paying approximately two-thirds of the public budget for health.

In 2003, donor funding for the health sector amounted to US$ 90 million, compared with an allocated government budget of 173 billion Riel (US$ 43.3 million) and only 167 billion Riel (US$ 41.8 million) disbursed.[18] This illustrates the importance of external funding for the health sector in Cambodia. External funding sources include United Nations agencies (20%); development banks (Asian Development Bank and World Bank) (6%); global initiatives, such as the Global Fund to Fight HIV/AIDS, Tuberculosis and Malaria (GFATM) (8%) and the Global Alliance for Vaccines and Immunization (GAVI) (1%); and bilateral (53%) and regional organizations such as the European Union (5%). The United States Agency for International Development (USAID) is by far the largest single external contributor to the health sector in Cambodia (32%)[19] (See Figure 10).

Figure 10: Coverage of child health survival packages

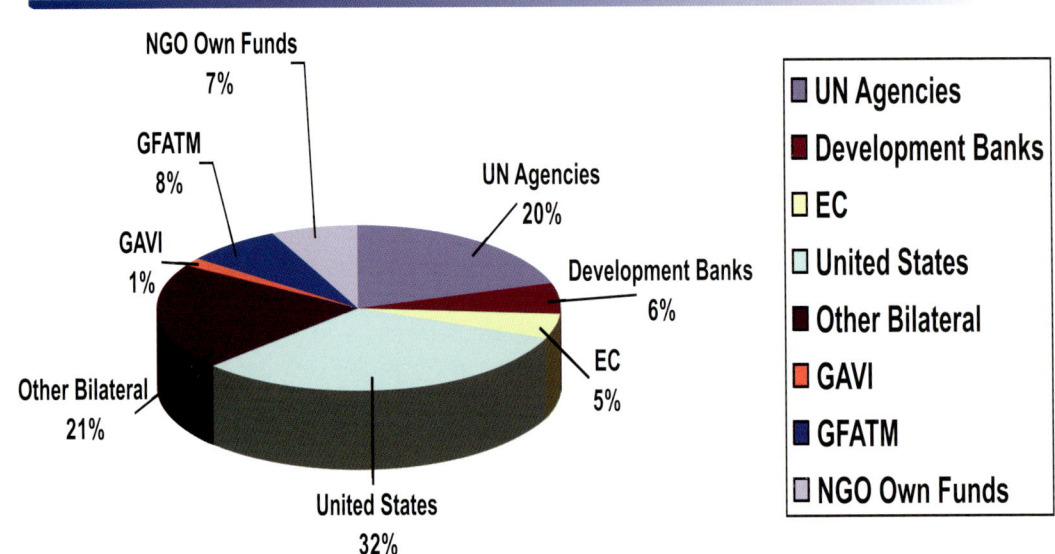

One quarter of all funds from external financing sources support the Maternal and Child Health (MCH), Safe Motherhood, Reproductive Health and Family Planning programmes (US$ 19.6 million). In comparison, US$ 29.3 million (35%) of donor funding is allocated to HIV/AIDS, and US$ 11.1 million (13%) to tuberculosis, malaria and dengue control programmes. Two-thirds of the MCH funds are for maternal and child health (US$ 13.3 million), including immunizations (US$ 1.7 million), and one-third for reproductive health, safe motherhood and family planning (US$ 6.3 million).[18]

As malaria and, to a lesser extent, HIV/AIDS affect children under five, funds devoted to those disease-specific control programmes also benefit child health, but it is not known to what extent the activities of the programmes benefit children under five years and at what cost. In general, the two diseases represent a minor contribution to child mortality. In addition, funds for health service delivery for children covered by Ministry of Health institutions outside programme budgets cannot be traced. In 2004, government funding for health was around US$ 56 million, but disbursement was low at 66% for recurrent costs and 49% for priority action programmes at district level. With the support of health development partners, the Ministry of Health is delivering a number of preventive child survival interventions to the population free of charge in outreach activities, including immunizations, the distribution of vitamin A capsules twice a year, and insecticide-treated bednets and their re-impregnation.

A Child Survival Costings Study[20] has been completed costing 11 of the 12 scorecard interventions with exception of skilled birth attendance which will be costed at a later date.

Table 9: Summary of scorecard intervention total commodity and program costs

Scorecard Interventions	2007	2008	2009	2010	Total 2007-10
Early initiation of breastfeeding	366,996	375,432	430,533	475,318	1,648,279
Exclusive breastfeeding	315,996	323,412	377,472	421,196	1,438,076
Complementary feeding	468,996	479,472	536,653	538,561	2,068,682
Vitamin A	1,538,133	1,587,611	1,651,816	1,727,444	6,505,004
Measles vaccine	2,980,337	1,801,723	1,813,421	1,771,458	8,366,939
Tetanus toxoid	2,882,390	2,663,185	2,669,287	2,529,534	10,744,396
Insecticide-treated nets (ITNs)	4,025,827	3,093,096	3,434,354	2,412,977	12,966,254
Malaria treatment	496,862	391,213	495,255	365,600	1,748,930
Dengue vector control	2,716,810	3,440,851	3,719,994	3,246,099	13,123,754
Oral rehydration theraphy (ORT)	2,914,834	3,141,545	3,594,266	3,923,760	13,574,405
Antibiotic for pneumonia	2,219,466	2,368,731	2,822,140	3,122,678	10,533,015
Skilled birth attendance	n/a	n/a	n/a	n/a	n/a
TOTAL	20,926,647	19,666,271	21,545,191	20,579,625	82,717,734

The costs do not include Ministry of Health staff and operating costs at the service delivery level or management level. Also some scorecard interventions include general activities for which the Reproductive Health Programme is responsible and these have not been costed. Covered in the study are the costs of implementing all the activities required under the interventions, and not the incremental costs of additional activities. The costs are spread fairly evenly over the four years from 2007 to 2010.

Curative care is provided by health centres while referral care is provided by national hospitals and by a large number of private providers. Up to 80% of health care expenditures comes from private sources, mainly out-of-pocket expenditure on curative care. The Health Financing Charter, established in 1996, allows public health facilities to charge patients for the services they provide.

The user-fee system provides income for the facilities, including some incentives for under paid health professionals. In 2004, user fees generated an income of US$ 6 million for the health sector, representing 4% of total health funding from all sources. Moreover, user fees may have improved the financial access of the population to the public health system, as they substantially reduce the unofficial fees charged to patients at the time of care. The user-fee system is complemented by exemption from fees for the most vulnerable members of the population. User fees are affordable at the health centre level and health centre staff are apparently more eager to grant exemptions to poor patients.[21] However, the cost of transport to public facilities remains an access barrier, particularly for the poor and populations living in remote or difficult-to-access areas.

At the hospital level, fees are higher and exemptions are not granted to all potential beneficiaries. The financial burden of transport, food and lodging is even higher. As a result, health expenditure for inpatient care represents a considerable financial risk for vulnerable populations. Catastrophic expenses for hospital care can tip families into extreme poverty.

For this reason, equity funds have been piloted in several operational districts since 2000. Equity funds identify poor households in the community, pay hospitals for the inpatient health care services provided to beneficiaries and reimburse the beneficiaries directly for additional costs such as transport and food. Equity funds cover all registered family members. Today, about twenty equity fund pilot projects exist.

In addition to equity funds, several community-based health insurance pilot projects have been initiated, also aimed at preventing households falling into extreme poverty. They target the near-poor population who can afford to pay a modest monthly premium in exchange of free health care at the time of delivery. Unlike equity funds, the community-based health insurance package includes primary as well as referral care. No information is available on the expenses for maternal and child health services covered by the initiatives.

The financial mechanisms described above aim to strengthen public health service delivery. However, the majority of the population seek health care in the private sector, mainly from unlicensed practitioners and drug sellers.[2] There is consistent evidence from anecdotal and qualitative research that, not only the choice of health care provider, but also the treatment sought by caretakers is often ill-informed. The private health care sector in Cambodia is still largely unregulated, and existing regulations are hardly enforced. No financial mechanism addresses the burden of health care costs in the sector, except a negligibly small private health insurance market for the better off. It is expected that strengthening public health service delivery, including aspects of financial access, will improve the confidence of patients in the public system and encourage them to modify their health-seeking behaviour. Social marketing approaches have been used to target the private sector to address mother and child health. Relevant to child survival are contraceptives, clean birth kits, artemisinine-based combination treatment for malaria (Malarine®, although this is not aimed at children under five), and ORS. A pilot study for the social marketing of a diarrhoea kit containing low osmolarity ORS and zinc tablets is under way. There is no information available on how many subsidies have gone into such programmes or how much the general public has spent on the commodities.

Charitable organizations play a significant role in financing health care for children, particularly hospital care. There are four NGO-run paediatric hospitals concentrated in the two major cities of Phnom Penh and Siem Reap. They provide free inpatient and outpatient health care services to children up to 15 years of age. The Kantha Bopha Hospital Foundation runs three of the paediatric hospitals. The NGO's own resources, i.e. those not provided by bilateral or other public sources, represent 7% of all external resources for the health sector.[18]

5. Collaboration and coordination

At national level, the newly established Child Survival Steering Committee, Management Committee and Executive Secretariat are responsible for the coordination of child survival activities. The members include programme managers from Communicable Disease Control, IMCI, National Immunization Programme, National Nutrition Programme, National Programme for Reproductive Health, National Centre for Health Promotion. Control of Diarrhoeal Disease/Acute Respiratory Illness, Dengue, Malaria and key partners. The National Maternal and Child Health Centre is also responsible for the coordination and implementation of both Safe Motherhood and other programmes related to child survival. There are programme managers for the Safe Motherhood, Immunization, Nutrition and Control of Diarrhoeal Diseases, Acute Respiratory Ilnesses and Cholera programmes.

Additionally, at the Ministry of Health level, several departments and programmes are related to child health interventions. These include: the Department for Communicable Disease Control, which hosts the Child Survival Executive Secretariat and the IMCI secretariat; the Department of Preventive Medicine; and the following national centres and programmes: the National Maternal and Child Health Centre (control of diarrhoeal disease, acute respiratory disease, immunization, nutrition, reproductive health programmes); the National Centre for Parasitology, Entomology and Malaria Control (programmes for control of malaria, dengue and intestinal parasites); and the National Centre for Health Promotion. The main clinical institutions at national level include the National Paediatric Hospital and the Kantha Bopha Foundation hospitals.

Coordination with partners is assured through the Technical Working Group for Health and its sub-committees, such as the MCH Coordination Sub-Committee and the Immunization Coordination Sub-Committee. The Child Survival Steering Committee will assist in this task related to child survival. For IMCI, the following coordination and managerial structures exist: an Advisory Committee, a Working Group with three sub-groups, and the IMCI secretariat. There are also specialized technical working groups dealing with micronutrients, infant and young child feeding, and immunizations.

The main issues related to the coordination and implementation of child health and nutrition programming include split responsibilities between many units, however, the Child Survival Management Committee is taking a strong role in encouraging technical coordination between departments and programmes, and improving lines of communication between the central-level Ministry of Health and the peripheral health authorities. At provincial and district levels the responsibilities for child health and nutrition will be coordinated through the newly designated Provincial Child Survival Management Committees.

Except for some national programmes, including the National Immunization and Nutrition programmes, and the national centres, budget allocations cannot be attributed specifically to child health, however annual operational plans of national programmes and provincial health departments should include budget line items for the 12 scorecard interventions which are already part of health services.

The Cambodian National Council for Children (CNCC) also has some mandate for child survival, however the involvement of this high-level body in health is limited, and its focus has been largely on other issues related to the Convention on the Rights of the Child (CRC). In addition, the Ministry of Health's involvement with the Council has also been limited. In 2003, the Technical Sub-Committee on Early Childhood Development was established with a mandate to coordinate and monitor the progress of interventions related to early childhood development. It also covers areas directly related to child survival, as listed in this report. Yet, the role of both the CNCC and the Sub-Committee is purely consultative, with no authority over any ministerial department and programme.

Other inter-ministerial bodies that have mandates related to the intervention areas covered in this report include: (1) the National Council for Nutrition, including the National Sub-Committee for the Control of Iodine Deficiency Disorders; (2) the Primary Health Care Inter- Ministerial Committee and Working Group; (3) the School Health Task Force of the Ministry of Education, Youth and Sports and the Ministry of Health; and (4) the IMCI Working Group, which also includes representatives of the Ministry of Rural Development, the Ministry of Education, Youth and Sports, and the Ministry of Women's and Veteran's Affairs. The mandates of these bodies often overlap and are not clearly delineated. They have proven to be useful for advocacy at higher political levels and for developing cross-sectoral policies and strategies, but they have had mixed results with regard to implementation and evaluating progress.

The formation of a strong central-level structure for child survival is now in place. The new structure facilitates the coordination of all partners working on child survival in Cambodia.

References

[1] *Cambodia inter-censal population survey 2004: general report.* Phnom Penh, Ministry of Planning, National Institute of Statistics, 2004.

[2] *Cambodia demographic and health survey 2005.* Phnom Penh, Ministry of Health, National Institute of Public Health: Ministry of Planning, National Institute of Statistics; Calverton, Md., ORC Macro, 2006.

[3] *1998 Census of Cambodia : report 7. Literarcy and education.* Phnom Penh, Ministry of Planning, National Institute of Statistics, 1998.

[4] *First revision population projections for Cambodia 1998-2020.* National Institute of Statistics, Ministry of Planning, 2004.

[5] *National accounts of Cambodia 1993-2005, bulletin no.10.* Phnom Penh, Ministry of Planning, National Institute of Statistics, 2006.

[6] *Human development report 2004 : cultural liberty in today's diverse world .* New York, UNDP, 2004.

[7] *Cambodia socio-economic survey 2004: summary subject matter report.* Phnom Penh, Ministry of Planning, National Institute of Statistics, 2005.

[8] *Cambodia: halving poverty by 2015?: poverty assessment 2006.* Washington, D.C., World Bank, 2006 .

[9] *Country health information profiles 2006.* Manila, WHO Western Pacific Regional Office, 2006.

[10] *Benchmark Report.* Phnom Penh, Ministry of Health Cambodia, 2005.

[11] *Cambodia Millennium Development Goals Report 2003.* Phnom Penh, Government of Cambodia, 2003.

[12] Cambodia. Council of Ministers. *National Strategic Development Plan 2006-2010.* Phnom Penh, Ministry of Planning, 2006.

[13] Jones G. *et al.* How many child deaths can we prevent this year? *Lancet* 2003, 362:65-71.

[14] Cambodia. Ministry of Health. National Maternal and Child Health Center. *National guidelines for the prevention of mother-to- child transmission of HIV. 2nd ed.* Phnom Penh, Ministry of Health, 2005.

[15] *Health sector strategic plan 2003-2007.* Phnom Penh, Ministry of Health, 2002 .

[16] The Development Study on Strengthening MCH Service Performance in the Kingdom of Cambodia, *Draft* Interim Report, 2006.

[17] Sherratt DR., White P., Chhuong CK. *Comprehensive midwifery review.* Phnom Penh, Council for the Development of Cambodia, Cambodian Rehabilitation and Development Board, 2006.

[18] *7th Consultative Group Meeting on Cambodia, Palais du Gouvernement, Phnom Penh, 6-7 December 2004: agenda and presentations.* Washington, D.C., The World Bank, 2004.

[19] Michaud CM. *External resource flows to the health sector in Cambodia.* Geneva, World Health Organization, 2005 . (WHO/SDE/CMH/05.2)

[20] Collins D., Lewis E., Stenberg K. *Scaling up child survival interventions in Cambodia : the cost of national programme resource needs: final report.* Geneva, World Health Organization, 2007.

[21] Wilkinson D ., Holloway J ., Fallavier P. *The impact of user fees on access, equity and health provider practices in Cambodia.* Phnom Penh, Ministry of Health, 2001.

Serviceteil

Sachregister – 237

Sachregister

A

Abduktion 137
Ad-hoc-Kompositum 100
Adstrate 173
Adverbial 84
Adverbialsatz 86
Affix **97**
Affixkonstanz 201
Akkusativobjekt 84
Akronym 101
Akzent 61
Akzeptabilität 7
Allograph 200
Allomorph **96**
Allophon 47
Ambiguität 121
Analogie 181
Anapher 153
Annotation **8**
Annotieren **8**
Antezedens 153
Antonymie 124
Aphasie 19
Argument 87
Argumentstruktur 87
Artikulationsmodus 35
Artikulationsort 34
Assimilation 51
Asterisk 18
Attribut 85
Attributsatz 86
Ausdrucksbedeutung 116
Äußerungsbedeutung 116
Autonomiehypothese 199

B

Basis **97**
Bedeutung 116
– deskriptive 119
– expressive 119
– soziale 119
Bedeutungsarten 116
Bedeutungsebenen 116
Bedeutungswandel 182
Broca-Aphasie 19
Buchstabe 198–201
Buchstabensegment 198

C

Computerlinguistik 19

D

Daten in der Linguistik 3, 6
Dativobjekt 84
Deduktion 137
Deiktischer Ausdruck 145
Deixis 145
– Lokaldeixis 145
– Personaldeixis 145
– Temporaldeixis 145
Deklination 80, 106
Denotation 115
Dependenzhypothese 199
Dependenztheorie *siehe* Dependenzhypothese
Derivation **101**, 104
Diakritikum 198
Dialekte
– primäre 167
– sekundäre 167
– tertiäre 167
Dialektometrie 169
Diffusion 187
Diglossie 172
Diphthong 58
Direktionale Opposition 124
Dissimilation 180
Distinktive Merkmale 53
Distribution 81

E

Elision 52
Ellipse 183
Empirische Linguistik **220**
Enchaînement 72
Entlehnung 184
Epenthese 52
Extension 114

F

Filter 142
Flexion 79, **100**
Flexionsdimension 99
Flexionseigenschaft *siehe* Flexionsdimension
Forschungsfrage 221
Frequenz 181
Fugenmorphem 98
Funktionale Priorität 199

G

Gender 17
Genderlinguistik 17
Genitivobjekt 84
Genus 80
Germanisch 18
Getrennt- und Zusammenschreibung 202
Glossierung 101
Glottis 29
GPK *siehe* Graphem-Phonem-Korrespondenz
Grammatikalisierung 186
Grammatikalitätsangaben **7**
Grammatischer Wandel 185
Graph 199, 200
Graphem 18, 199, **200**
– komplexes 200, 201
Graphematik 18, **198**
– Deutsch 204
– romanische Sprachen 205
– suprasegmentale 201

Graphematische Hierarchie 199
Graphem-Phonem-Korrespondenz 200
Graphotaktik 203
Großschreibung 203

H

Hauptsatz 85
Hiatus 58
Historische Linguistik 17
Homografievermeidung *siehe* Lexemdifferenzierung
Homographie 122
Homonymie 122
– partielle 122
– vollständige 122
Homophonie 122
Hyperonymie 123
Hyponymie 123
Hypothese **221**

I

Illokutionärer Indikator 147
Implikatur 135
– konventionelle 138
– konversationelle 139
– konversationelle generalisierte 139
– konversationelle partikularisierte 139
– skalare 139
Indirekter Sprechakt 147
Induktion 137
Infix **98**
Innovation 187
Intension 114
Interdependenzhypothese 199
Interdependenztheorie *siehe* Interdependenzhypothese
Interlinearglosse 103
Internationales Phonetisches Alphabet 44
Interpunktionszeichen 198, 203
Intertextualität 154
Intonation 63
Introspektion **7**
IPA 44
Isoglosse 168

K

Kardinalvokale 38
Kasus 80
Klitische Verschmelzung 102
Koda 56
Kohärenz 153
Kohäsion 153
Kommunikativer Sinn 118
Komparation 80, 106
Kompetenz **11**, 13
Komplementarität 124
Komposition **100**, 103, 107
Kompositionalitätsprinzip 125
Konjugation 80, 106
Konnotation 119
Konsonant 32, 34, 44
Konstituente 77, 82
Kontinuum 166
Konversationsmaximen 136
Konversion **100**
Konzept 113

Kooperativitätsprinzip 136
Koordinationstest 83
Kopf 83
Korpus 6, **7**, **221**
Korpuslinguistik **226**
Korpustypen **10**
Kriterien für Textualität 153
Kurzwortbildung **101**

L

Lambda-Kalkül 126
Langue 13
Larynx 28
Lautwandel 180
Leipzig glossing rules 103
Lexem **98**
Lexemdifferenzierung 202
Lexikalische Relation 123
Liaison 72
Löcher 142
Logik 135

M

Maschinelle Übersetzung 20
Matrixsatz 86
Merkmalgeometrie 67
Metadaten 8
Metapher 182
Metasprache 101
Metonymie 122, 183
Minimalpaar 199
Modalität 129
Modus 80, 129
Monophthong 58
Morph **96**
Morphem **96**
– freies **97**
– gebundenes **97**
Morphemkonstanz 200, **201**
Morphemschrift *siehe* Schriftsysteme
Morphologie 12, **14**, **94**, 200
– konkatenative 103
– nicht-konkatenative 103
Morphologische Reanalyse 182
Morphologischer Wandel 181
Morphophonologische Alternation **106**

N

Natürliche Klasse 53
Natürlichkeitstheorie 190
Nebensatz 85
Negation 127
Neologismus 94
Neurolinguistik 19
Notationskonventionen
– Graphematik **200**
Nukleus 56
Nullmorphem 96, **101**
Numerus 80

O

Objektsatz 86
Objektsprache 101

Onset 56
Ontogenetische Priorität 199
Optimalitätstheorie 69
Orthografie **198**

P

Paradigma **99**
Paradigmatische Nivellierung 182
Parole 13
Partikel 106
Performanz **11**, 13
Performative Äußerung 146
Person 80
PGK *siehe* Phonem-Graphem-Korrespondenz
Phonem 46
Phonem-Graphem-Korrespondenz 200
Phonetik **12**
– akustische 27, 39
– artikulatorische 27, 28
– perzeptive 27, 42
Phonologie **12**, 46, 106, 199
– autosegmentale 65
Phonologische Alternationen 50
Phrase 83
Phylogenetische Priorität 199
Polysemie 122
Präfix **97**
Pragmatik 15, **16**
Präpositionalobjekt 84
Präsupposition 135, 140
Präsuppositionsauslöser 142
Präsuppositionsprojektion 142
Primärdaten 8
Produktivität 181
Proposition 125
Propositionaler Gehalt 125
Prototyp 115
Psycholinguistik 19, **228**

Q

Quantifikation 128
Quantor 128

R

Raddoppiamento Sintattico 72
Raumausdrücke 128
Reanalyse 185
Referenz 113, 143
Referenzkette 155
Referierender Ausdruck 143
Reim 56
Rekonstruktion von Verwandtschaftsverhältnissen 179
Rektion 81
Relativsatz 86

S

Sandhi 70
Satz 77
Satzakzent 61
Satzart 88
Satzbedeutung 15
Satzglied 84
Satztyp 88

Satzzeichen *siehe* Interpunktionszeichen
de Saussure, Ferdinand 13
Schibboleth 171
Schluss
– logischer 134
– pragmatischer 136
Schreibsilbe 201
Schriftsysteme 198
– alphabetische 198
– Morphemschrift 198
– phonemische 198
– Silbenschrift 198
Semantik **15**
Semantische Rollen 88
Semasiographisches Zeichen 198
Semiotisches Dreieck 115
Silbe 56
– graphematische 201
– phonologische 201
Silbengelenkschreibung 200
Silbeninitiales <h> 203
Silbenkern 56
Silbenschrift *siehe* Schriftsysteme
Sonorität 59
Soziolinguistik 16
Spracheinstellungsforschung 171
Sprachgeschichte
– externe 178
– interne 178
Sprachliche Variation 162
Sprachpflege 3
Sprachstufen 18
Sprachvergleich 130, 148
Sprachwandelmodelle
– organizistische 188
– strukturalistische 189
Sprachwandeltheorien 179
– mentalistische 192
– sozio-kulturelle 191
Sprechakt 146
– Äußerungsakt 146
– illokutionärer Akt 146
– perlokutionärer Akt 146
– propositionaler Akt 146
Stammalternation 103
Stammkonstanz 201
Standardsprachen 166
Stelligkeit 14
Stöpsel 142
Strukturelle Priorität 199
STTS *siehe* Stuttgart-Tübingen Tagset
Stuttgart-Tübingen Tagset 8
Subjekt 84
Subjektsatz 86
Substitutionstest 83
Substrate 173
Suffix **97**
Superstrate 173
Synekdoche 183
Synonymie 123
Syntax 14, **15**, 76, 105, 203

T

Tag **8**
Tagset **8**

Tempus   80, 129
Text   16, 152
Textlinguistik   16, 152
Textsorte   156
Ton   66
Tonsprache   66
Topologie   89
Transkription   6
Type   **224**

U

Umlaut   106
Umstellungstest   83
Universalgrammatik   192

V

Variation
– diaphasische   163
– diastratische   163
– diatopische   163
Varietät, sprachliche   164
Varietätenkette   164
Varietätenlinguistik   16

Velum   28
Verb
– schwach   106
– stark   106
Vokal   32, 36, 44
Vokaltrakt   27
Vokaltrapez   38
Volksetymologie   184

W

Wernicke-Aphasie   19
Wort   77, 102
Wortakzent   29, 61
Wortarten   79
Wortbedeutung   15
Wortbildung   13, 101
Worterkennung   12
Wortform   **98**
Wurzel   **97**

Z

Zeit   129
Zirkumfix   **98**

The manufacturer's authorised representative in the EU is Springer Nature Customer Service Centre GmbH, Europaplatz 3, 69115 Heidelberg, Germany. If you have any concerns regarding our products, please contact ProductSafety@springernature.com

Printed and bound by CPI Group (UK) Ltd, Croydon, CR0 4YY
23/03/2026
02076403-0001